Pain Relief with Natural Salves

30 Homemade Recipes

Table of Contents

Introduction 5

Chapter 1. An Overview of Herbal Remedies 6

Chapter 2. Essential Oil & Herb Recipes for Natural Pain Relief 9
   1. Goodness in the Air... 9
   2. Air Filled with Bliss 10
   3. Feeling In a Good Mood 11
   4. Soother of Sore Throat 12
   5. Flu Attacker.. 13
   6. Choice of Athlete's 14
   7. Total Motion Blend 15
   8. Dancing for Joy 16
   9. Stiffness No More 17
   10. Tamer of Tummy Ache.. 18
   11. Free Movement 19
   12. Glee Days 20
   13. Special Muscle Magic... 21
   14. Magic Back Booster.. 22
   15. Headache Melter 23
   16. Healthy Joints... 24
   17. Worry Melter.. 25
   18. Staying Tuned-In.. 26
   19. Immediate Burn Relief... 27
   20. Feeling Young Again 28

Chapter 3. Herbal Teas & Tonics.. 29
   21. All Is Good... 29
   22. Guys and Gals 30
   23. Peachy Keen Longevity 31
   24. Mighty Apple 32

25. Tea Tonic for Rest.. 33

26. Achy Breaky Mix... 34

27. Super Hero for Fighting Cold & Flu.. 35

28. Sore Throat Eliminator.. 36

29. Soother of Stomach.. 37

30. Feeling Lively 38

Conclusion 39

FREE Bonus Reminder 40

Introduction

I would first like to thank and congratulate you on downloading *"Homemade Salves for Pain Relief."* Just by downloading this book it shows that you are truly serious about preparing your own natural home remedies. I can assure you that you will feel so much better just in knowing that the remedies you are going to use are all natural and are not filled with harmful chemicals or additives. More and more people are searching for healthier and more natural selections in many different areas from the food choices we make to the products that we are using on our skin to help keep it looking and feeling healthy.

You can feel good when you are using natural products in and on your body. You want to make sure that you are making the best choices when it comes to treating your body and its ailments. Using natural remedies are the best way to ensure that you are doing what is best for your body without compromising the rest of your health.

I am sure you have hesitations about turning to natural remedies. In this book I will show you how you can use essential oils and herbs effectively, getting the results that you seek without emptying your bank to do so. By introducing you to the world of herbs and oils through this book I hope that we can have you feeling like your old self in no time. When it comes to choosing synthetic remedies over natural remedies—natural is always the better and healthier choice!

You will find the collection of remedies in this book very simple and easy to follow and prepare. When you are purchasing your essential oils I would suggest going to a health food store that sells quality items. In this store you should look for the essential oils that are in dark glass bottles and are said to be therapeutic grade and 100% pure essential oils. You have to be on the look out for those trying to sell watered down or essential oils that have other things added to them. To help you with your treatments of ailments you want to make sure that you are using the therapeutic grade essential oils. Make sure when storing them to keep them in a dark and cool place. Once you have acquired a diffuser and essential oils you have the basics to begin starting your natural treatments of your ailments. Using herbal remedies is certainly not something that is new to mankind, but indeed they have been around for hundreds of years long before modern medicine was in the picture. Now many of us are turning back to our herbal remedy roots and seeking a more healthy and natural way to heal our ailments using essential oils and herbs.

Chapter 1. An Overview of Herbal Remedies

Herbs have been used to treat a plethora of ailments long before modern medicine ever entered the picture. You can find herbs to relieve symptoms from headaches, joint aches and muscle cramps, resulting in you getting back on your feet in no time.

However, I must point out that not all herbs are the same, it is important that you are aware of what you are using in your treatments. Some herbs will have a more pleasant taste than others, become familiar with what herbs you need to use to treat certain ailments. In this book I will help show you how to use both herbs and essential oils in ways I am sure you haven't before. I will show you how you can treat a number of illnesses and health problems, using natural remedies and you won't have to step inside a doctor's office to do it.

I will show you how you can use aromatherapy and teas to treat your body aches and pains, and how to use herbs to achieve the same health benefits that expensive medications provide without the side effects often accompanied with synthetic medications.

Of course when you are taking your herbal remedies you still must exercise moderation, but you will not have to worry about a long list of symptoms when you take herbal remedies, because they are safe to use.

What you do need to learn is what herbs you need to use to treat the health condition you are facing. You can often make a nice tea from herbs that can soon have you feeling back to your old self in no time. You will be able to effectively treat ailments from mild aches and pains to pains you feel from age or those caused from an illness with herbs and essential oils.

Through the use of homemade remedies you can rid yourself of the aches and pains you have been facing on a daily basis, and get back to your old self in no time!

Aromatherapy

When it comes to using essential oils for helping to heal and improve your health and well-being you simply can't go wrong. These oils have been in use for hundreds of years, helping to heal and treat many different ailments with their healing powers.

An essential oil is a concentrated oil that is derived from plants. Most often they are extracted from the leaves and fruits of various plants, but they can also come from the roots and seeds of plants.

When choosing essential oils for your health, you want to make sure to choose oils that are 100% pure essential oils. Look on the bottle for the words "therapy grade" and "100% pure" when shopping for your essential oils, make sure that they come in dark bottles as well. In order for essential oils to remain potent they must be stored in dark bottles. If you find essential oils that are not in a dark bottle they are more than likely not going to be pure essential oils.

You will need to choose a diffuser to practice the use of aromatherapy. You can purchase a wide array of different styles of diffusers online. There are literally dozens of styles and materials in diffusers for you to choose from, find one that suits your taste and decor. Depending on the size of diffuser you get you can run it for 12 hours. The smaller tanks run about 2 to 4 hours, choose a size that will suit your needs.

How effective is aromatherapy?

There has been many different studies that have shown aromatherapy to be just as effective as conventional medicine when it comes to treating an assortment of ailments. People that found it difficult to focus have said that they noticed an improvement when using aromatherapy, finding that their minds seemed sharper.

Using aromatherapy can help to relieve headaches, anxiety, depression as well as other ailments. When you mix essential oils with a carrier oil and apply them to your skin they have been proven to be very effective.

Use essential oils in the treatment of muscle cramps, joint aches, and even stomachaches along with many other ailments.

Can you overdose on essential oils?

There are many people that debate on whether essential oils are safe to ingest, I would suggest not ingest them just to play it safe so to speak. If you use them in your diffuser as instructed then there is no worry of overdosing on the essential oils.

However, if you are applying the essential oils directly to your skin then you need to first mix them with a carrier oil. You need to use a carrier oil as they are highly concentrated and could cause skin irritation if applied without mixing with carrier oil first. Make sure that you keep your essential oils out of the reach of children.

Overall I am sure that you are going to just love using essential oils and aromatherapy!

Chapter 2. Essential Oil & Herb Recipes for Natural Pain Relief

For many of these recipes blends you can use a diffuser, allowing the healthy goodness to fill the air around you. However, for direct application you need to blend the essential oils with a carrier oil and massage externally into the affected area. Do not ingest the essential oils.

1. Goodness in the Air

Ingredients:

- 5 drops rose essential oil

- 10 drops chamomile essential oil

- 10 drops lavender essential oil

Directions:

If you are using a diffuser, place these essential oils into a jar and shake well to combine them.   After combining the oils transfer them to the diffuser, filling it with water according to the instructions of your diffuser. Plug in your diffuser and allow the aromatherapy to take affect, offering you the relief that you are seeking.

To apply directly, mix oils in jar then add in 2 tablespoons of coconut oil and massage into the affected area. Repeat this morning and night as needed.

2. Air Filled with Bliss

Ingredients:

- 10 drops of vanilla essential oil

- 10 drops of sunflower essential oil

- 8 drops of geranium essential oil

Directions:

First you want to combine your essential oils in a jar and shake well. Transfer the mixed oils into the diffuser, fill with water according to your diffuser instructions. Turn on your diffuser and breath in that healing air.

For direct application, combine oils in jar and shake well, add in 2 tablespoons of coconut oil and massage into the affected area. Repeat this process morning and night as needed.

3. *Feeling In a Good Mood*

Ingredients:

- 10 drops chamomile essential oil

- 10 drops myrrh essential oil

- 10 drops lavender essential oil

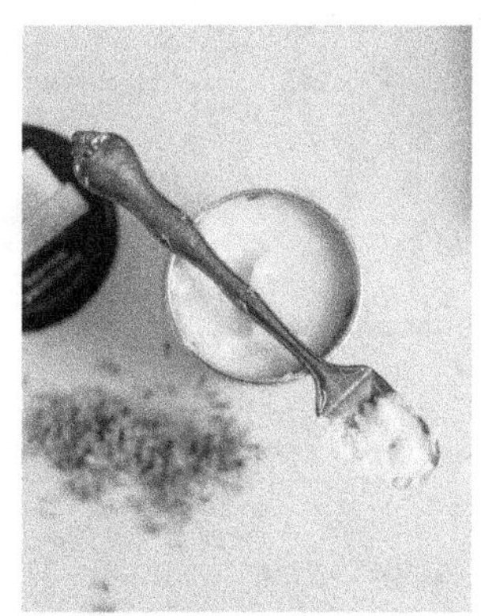

Directions:

First you want to combine your essential oils in a jar and shake well. Transfer the mixed oils into the diffuser, fill with water according to your diffuser instructions. Turn on your diffuser and breath in that healing air.

For direct application, combine oils in jar and shake well, add in 2 tablespoons of coconut oil and massage into the affected area. Repeat this process morning and night as needed.

4. Soother of Sore Throat

Ingredients:

- 12 drops peppermint essential oil

- 12 drops cinnamon essential oil

Directions:

First you want to combine your essential oils in a jar and shake well. Transfer the mixed oils into the diffuser, fill with water according to your diffuser instructions. Turn on your diffuser and breath in that healing air.

For direct application, combine oils in jar and shake well, add in 2 tablespoons of coconut oil and massage into the affected area. Repeat this process morning and night as needed.

5. Flu Attacker

Ingredients:

- 10 drops ginger essential oil

- 10 drops cinnamon essential oil

- 8 drops blood orange essential oil

Directions:

First you want to combine your essential oils in a jar and shake well. Transfer the mixed oils into the diffuser, fill with water according to your diffuser instructions. Turn on your diffuser and breath in that healing air.

For direct application, combine oils in jar and shake well, add in 2 tablespoons of coconut oil and massage into the affected area. Repeat this process morning and night as needed.

6. Choice of Athlete's

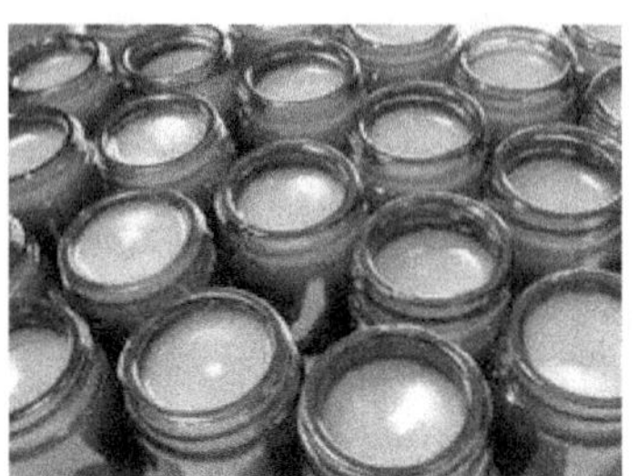

Ingredients:

- 8 drops peppermint essential oil

- 8 drops rosewood essential oil

- 10 drops rose essential oil

Directions:

First you want to combine your essential oils in a jar and shake well. Transfer the mixed oils into the diffuser, fill with water according to your diffuser instructions. Turn on your diffuser and breath in that healing air.

For direct application, combine oils in jar and shake well, add in 2 tablespoons of coconut oil and massage into the affected area. Repeat this process morning and night as needed.

7. Total Motion Blend

Ingredients:

- 8 drops of patchouli essential oil

- 8 drops of basil essential oil

- 10 drops of cinnamon essential oil

Directions:

First you want to combine your essential oils in a jar and shake well. Transfer the mixed oils into the diffuser, fill with water according to your diffuser instructions. Turn on your diffuser and breath in that healing air.

For direct application, combine oils in jar and shake well, add in 2 tablespoons of coconut oil and massage into the affected area. Repeat this process morning and night as needed.

8. Dancing for Joy

Ingredients:

- 5 drops of fir needle essential oil

- 8 drops of tea tree essential oil

- 10 drops of grapefruit essential oil

Directions:

First you want to combine your essential oils in a jar and shake well. Transfer the mixed oils into the diffuser, fill with water according to your diffuser instructions. Turn on your diffuser and breath in that healing air.

For direct application, combine oils in jar and shake well, add in 2 tablespoons of coconut oil and massage into the affected area. Repeat this process morning and night as needed.

9. Stiffness No More

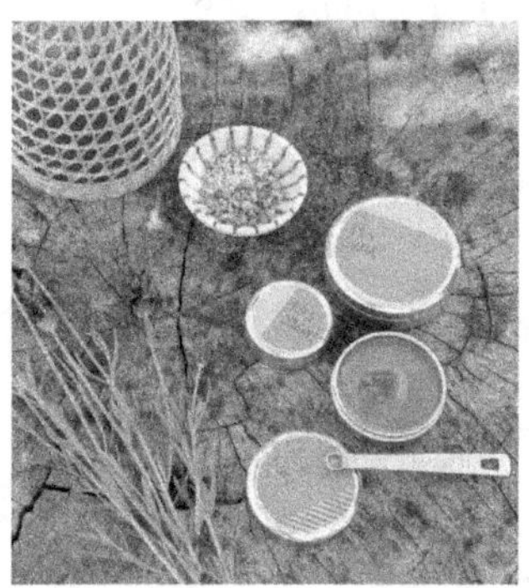

Ingredients:

- 8 drops of myrrh essential oil

- 8 drops of tea tree essential oil

- 12 drops of geranium essential oil

Directions:

First you want to combine your essential oils in a jar and shake well. Transfer the mixed oils into the diffuser, fill with water according to your diffuser instructions. Turn on your diffuser and breath in that healing air.

For direct application, combine oils in jar and shake well, add in 2 tablespoons of coconut oil and massage into the affected area. Repeat this process morning and night as needed.

10. *Tamer of Tummy Ache*

Ingredients:

- 5 drops eucalyptus essential oil

- 12 drops ginger essential oil

- 12 drops peppermint essential oil

Directions:

First you want to combine your essential oils in a jar and shake well. Transfer the mixed oils into the diffuser, fill with water according to your diffuser instructions. Turn on your diffuser and breath in that healing air.

For direct application, combine oils in jar and shake well, add in 2 tablespoons of coconut oil and massage into the affected area. Repeat this process morning and night as needed.

11. Free Movement

Ingredients:

- 9 drops of sandalwood essential oil

- 9 drops of Goldenseal essential oil

- 12 drops of myrrh essential oil

Directions:

First you want to combine your essential oils in a jar and shake well. Transfer the mixed oils into the diffuser, fill with water according to your diffuser instructions. Turn on your diffuser and breath in that healing air.

For direct application, combine oils in jar and shake well, add in 2 tablespoons of coconut oil and massage into the affected area. Repeat this process morning and night as needed.

12. Glee Days

Ingredients:

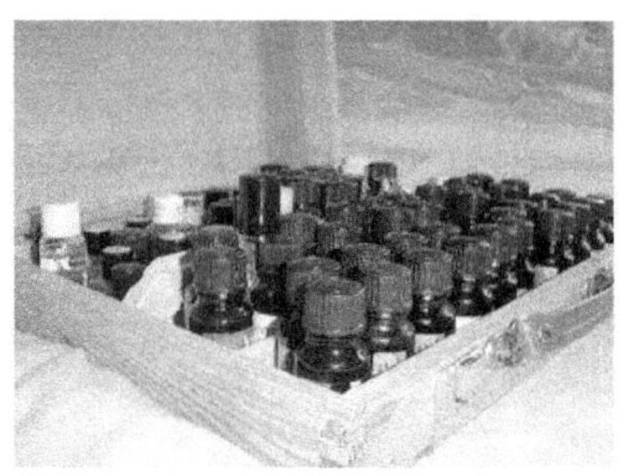

- 8 drops of lemon essential oil

- 8 drops of lavender essential oil

- 12 drops of chamomile essential oil

Directions:

First you want to combine your essential oils in a jar and shake well. Transfer the mixed oils into the diffuser, fill with water according to your diffuser instructions. Turn on your diffuser and breath in that healing air.

For direct application, combine oils in jar and shake well, add in 2 tablespoons of coconut oil and massage into the affected area. Repeat this process morning and night as needed.

13. Special Muscle Magic

Ingredients:

- 8 drops of lemon essential oil

- 8 drops of cinnamon essential oil

- 12 drops of grapefruit essential oil

Directions:

First you want to combine your essential oils in a jar and shake well. Transfer the mixed oils into the diffuser, fill with water according to your diffuser instructions. Turn on your diffuser and breath in that healing air.

For direct application, combine oils in jar and shake well, add in 2 tablespoons of coconut oil and massage into the affected area. Repeat this process morning and night as needed.

14. Magic Back Booster

Ingredients:

- 8 drops of blood orange essential oil

- 12 drops of Frankincense essential oil

- 8 drops of lemon essential oil

Directions:

First you want to combine your essential oils in a jar and shake well. Transfer the mixed oils into the diffuser, fill with water according to your diffuser instructions. Turn on your diffuser and breath in that healing air.

For direct application, combine oils in jar and shake well, add in 2 tablespoons of coconut oil and massage into the affected area. Repeat this process morning and night as needed.

15. Headache Melter

Ingredients:

- 8 drops of ginger essential oil

- 8 drops of geranium essential oil

- 12 drops of peppermint essential oil

Directions:

First you want to combine your essential oils in a jar and shake well. Transfer the mixed oils into the diffuser, fill with water according to your diffuser instructions. Turn on your diffuser and breath in that healing air.

For direct application, combine oils in jar and shake well, add in 2 tablespoons of coconut oil and massage into the affected area. Repeat this process morning and night as needed.

16. Healthy Joints

Ingredients:

- 10 drops of myrrh essential oil

- 10 drops of Frankincense essential oil

- 8 drops of cinnamon essential oil

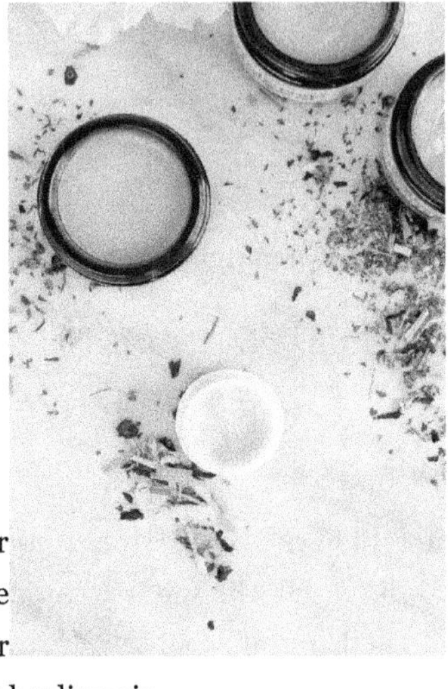

Directions:

First you want to combine your essential oils in a jar and shake well. Transfer the mixed oils into the diffuser, fill with water according to your diffuser instructions. Turn on your diffuser and breath in that healing air.

For direct application, combine oils in jar and shake well, add in 2 tablespoons of coconut oil and massage into the affected area. Repeat this process morning and night as needed.

17. Worry Melter

Ingredients:

- 9 drops of lemon essential oil

- 9 drops of lavender essential oil

- 12 drops of peppermint essential oil

Directions:

First you want to combine your essential oils in a jar and shake well. Transfer the mixed oils into the diffuser, fill with water according to your diffuser instructions. Turn on your diffuser and breath in that healing air.

For direct application, combine oils in jar and shake well, add in 2 tablespoons of coconut oil and massage into the affected area. Repeat this process morning and night as needed.

18. Staying Tuned-In

Ingredients:

- 9 drops of eucalyptus essential oil

- 9 drops of spearmint essential oil

- 12 drops of peppermint essential oil

Directions:

First you want to combine your essential oils in a jar and shake well. Transfer the mixed oils into the diffuser, fill with water according to your diffuser instructions. Turn on your diffuser and breath in that healing air.

For direct application, combine oils in jar and shake well, add in 2 tablespoons of coconut oil and massage into the affected area. Repeat this process morning and night as needed.

19. Immediate Burn Relief

Ingredients:

- 12 drops of myrrh essential oil

- 8 drops eucalyptus essential oil

Directions:

First you want to combine your essential oils in a jar and shake well. Transfer the mixed oils into the diffuser, fill with water according to your diffuser instructions. Turn on your diffuser and breath in that healing air.

For direct application, combine oils in jar and shake well, add in 2 tablespoons of coconut oil and massage into the affected area. Repeat this process morning and night as needed.

20. Feeling Young Again

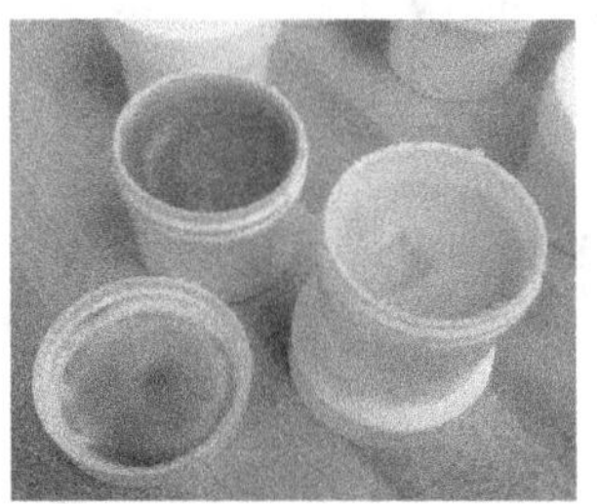

Ingredients:

- 12 drops of vanilla essential oil

- 10 drops of myrrh essential oil

Directions:

First you want to combine your essential oils in a jar and shake well. Transfer the mixed oils into the diffuser, fill with water according to your diffuser instructions. Turn on your diffuser and breath in that healing air.

For direct application, combine oils in jar and shake well, add in 2 tablespoons of coconut oil and massage into the affected area. Repeat this process morning and night as needed.

Chapter 3. Herbal Teas & Tonics

To help to give you that extra boost from time to time I would suggest using herbal teas and tonics. Using herbal remedies is something that mankind has been using for hundreds of years and is still used today in spite of modern medicine. Use these wonderful blends to help get you back to your old self in no time—without any harmful side effects.

21. *All Is Good*

Ingredients:

- 2 teaspoons black tea leaves

- 1 teaspoon turmeric root

- 1 teaspoon ginger root

- 2 teaspoons raspberry leaves

- 2 teaspoons of ginseng leaves

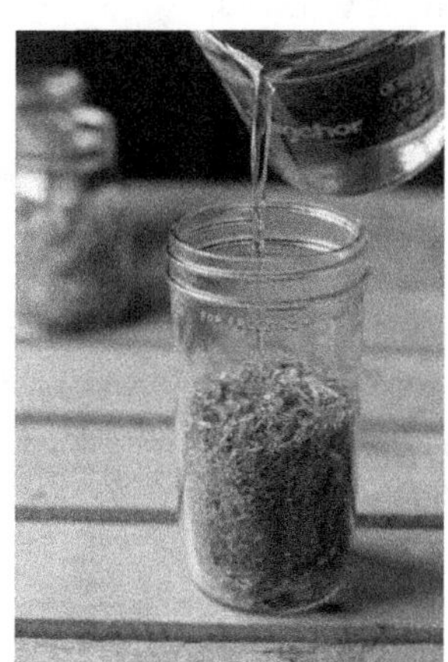

Directions:

Make sure that all of the leaves are broken down into small bits. Place them into a tea ball or inside tea paper. Fill your mug with hot water, then place in the tea blend. Allow it to steep for a good 5 minutes before you drink it. I would recommend leaving the ball in the water for a good 15 minutes. Enjoy a nice glass of tea in the morning and late afternoon, or whenever you feel the need for an extra boost.

22. Guys and Gals

Ingredients:

- 2 teaspoons black tea leaves

- 2 teaspoons rosehip, ground

- 1 teaspoon of raspberry leaves

- honey to taste

Directions:

Make sure that all of the leaves are broken down into small bits. Place them into a tea ball or inside tea paper. Fill your mug with hot water, then place in the tea blend. Allow it to steep for a good 5 minutes before you drink it. I would recommend leaving the ball in the water for a good 15 minutes. Enjoy a nice glass of tea in the morning and late afternoon, or whenever you feel the need for an extra boost.

23. Peachy Keen Longevity

Ingredients:

- 1 teaspoon of ginger root

- 2 teaspoons of peach pit, ground

- 2 teaspoons of black tea leaves

- honey to taste

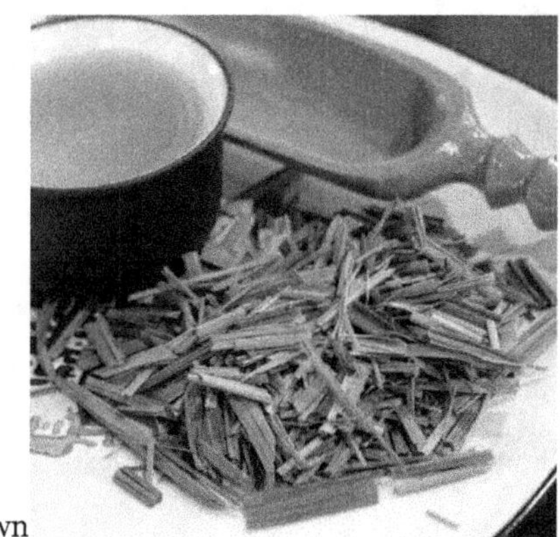

Directions:

Make sure that all of the leaves are broken down into small bits. Place them into a tea ball or inside tea paper. Fill your mug with hot water, then place in the tea blend. Allow it to steep for a good 5 minutes before you drink it. I would recommend leaving the ball in the water for a good 15 minutes. Enjoy a nice glass of tea in the morning and late afternoon, or whenever you feel the need for an extra boost.

24. Mighty Apple

Ingredients:

- 1 teaspoon of cinnamon bark

- 1 tablespoon of apple cider vinegar

- 1 tablespoon of apples, dehydrated

- 1 teaspoon of ginger, ground

- 2 teaspoons of black tea leaves

- honey to taste

Directions:

Make sure that all of the leaves are broken down into small bits. Place them into a tea ball or inside tea paper. Fill your mug with hot water, then place in the tea blend. Allow it to steep for a good 5 minutes before you drink it. I would recommend leaving the ball in the water for a good 15 minutes. Enjoy a nice glass of tea in the morning and late afternoon, or whenever you feel the need for an extra boost.

25. Tea Tonic for Rest

Ingredients:

- 2 teaspoons of black tea leaves

- 1 teaspoon of chamomile leaves

- 1 teaspoon of Valerian root

- honey to taste

Directions:

Make sure that all of the leaves are broken down into small bits. Place them into a tea ball or inside tea paper. Fill your mug with hot water, then place in the tea blend. Allow it to steep for a good 5 minutes before you drink it. I would recommend leaving the ball in the water for a good 15 minutes. Enjoy a nice glass of tea in the morning and late afternoon, or whenever you feel the need for an extra boost.

Ingredients:

- 2 teaspoons of black tea leaves

- 2 teaspoons of ginseng leaves

- 1 teaspoon of St. John's Wort leaves

- honey to taste

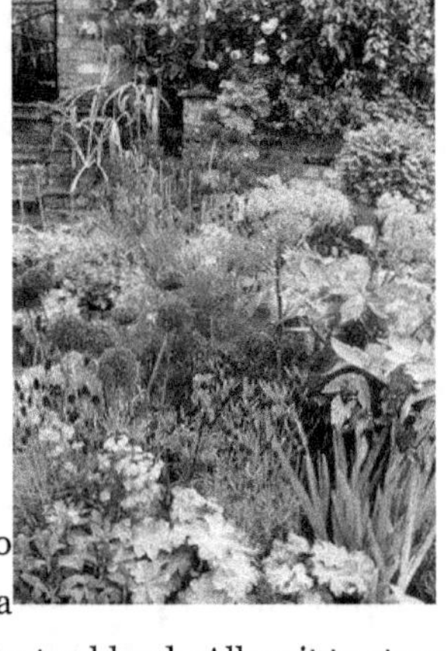

Directions:

Make sure that all of the leaves are broken down into small bits. Place them into a tea ball or inside tea paper. Fill your mug with hot water, then place in the tea blend. Allow it to steep for a good 5 minutes before you drink it. I would recommend leaving the ball in the water for a good 15 minutes. Enjoy a nice glass of tea in the morning and late afternoon, or whenever you feel the need for an extra boost.

27. Super Hero for Fighting Cold & Flu

Ingredients:

- 2 teaspoons black tea leaves

- 1 teaspoon of mint leaves

- 1 teaspoon marshmallow leaves, ground

- 1 tablespoon organic lemon peel, dried

Directions:

Make sure that all of the leaves are broken down into small bits. Place them into a tea ball or inside tea paper. Fill your mug with hot water, then place in the tea blend. Allow it to steep for a good 5 minutes before you drink it. I would recommend leaving the ball in the water for a good 15 minutes. Enjoy a nice glass of tea in the morning and late afternoon, or whenever you feel the need for an extra boost.

28. Sore Throat Eliminator

Ingredients:

- 2 teaspoons of black tea leaves

- 1 teaspoon of licorice root

- 1/4 teaspoon cayenne pepper

- honey to taste

Directions:

Make sure that all of the leaves are broken down into small bits. Place them into a tea ball or inside tea paper. Fill your mug with hot water, then place in the tea blend. Allow it to steep for a good 5 minutes before you drink it. I would recommend leaving the ball in the water for a good 15 minutes. Enjoy a nice glass of tea in the morning and late afternoon, or whenever you feel the need for an extra boost.

29. Soother of Stomach

Ingredients:

- 1 teaspoon of ginger root, chopped

- 2 teaspoons black tea leaves

- 2 teaspoons peppermint leaves

- honey to taste

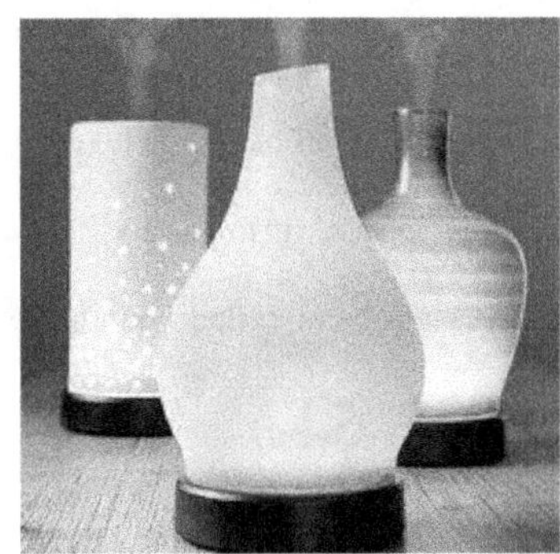

Directions:

Make sure that all of the leaves are broken down into small bits. Place them into a tea ball or inside tea paper. Fill your mug with hot water, then place in the tea blend. Allow it to steep for a good 5 minutes before you drink it. I would recommend leaving the ball in the water for a good 15 minutes. Enjoy a nice glass of tea in the morning and late afternoon, or whenever you feel the need for an extra boost.

30. Feeling Lively

Ingredients:

- 2 teaspoons of black tea leaves

- 1 teaspoon of turmeric root, chopped

- 2 teaspoons of ginger root, chopped

- honey to taste

Directions:

Make sure that all of the leaves are broken down into small bits. Place them into a tea ball or inside tea paper. Fill your mug with hot water, then place in the tea blend. Allow it to steep for a good 5 minutes before you drink it. I would recommend leaving the ball in the water for a good 15 minutes. Enjoy a nice glass of tea in the morning and late afternoon, or whenever you feel the need for an extra boost.

Conclusion

I hope that you and your loved ones will benefit from using the recipes in this book to help to ease your aches and pains in a natural and healthy way that will not include any harmful side effects and not cost a fortune. Feel good in knowing that you can easily and inexpensively prepare these remedies up for yourself and loved ones. Choosing to use natural remedies to ease your aches and pains is definitely a smart and healthy choice. In this fast paced world that we live in today many more people are searching for more simple and wholesome remedies to get them feeling right as rain again. People are looking for remedies for ailments that are not accompanied with severe side effects like many synthetic medications have. Many of us are realizing that the natural choice is the more healthy choice when choosing a kind of treatment for our ailments. Of course it is always good to talk with your physician about any treatments that you are considering. It is always better to be safe than sorry, so make sure that you have the thumbs up from your medical care provider before starting any new form of treatment.

I would like to thank you once again for downloading my book and supporting my work. I cannot begin to tell you how much your support means to me. I would love to read a review by you of my book on Amazon. Take care and best of luck at trying out my collection of essential oil and herb remedies for aches and pains.

FREE Bonus Reminder

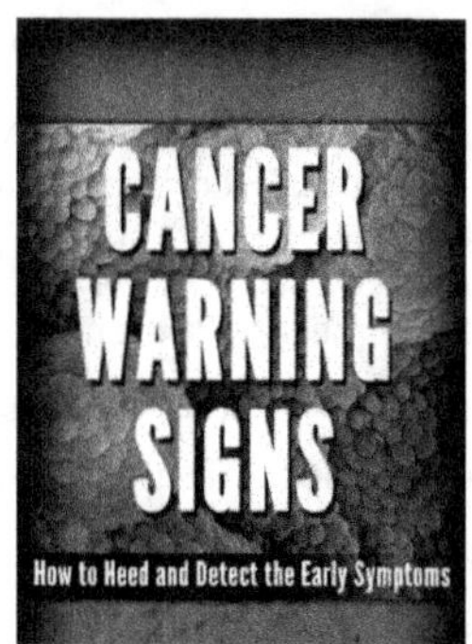

If you have not grabbed it yet, please go ahead and download your special bonus report *"Cancer Warning Signs. How To Heed & Detect The Early Symptoms!"*
Simply Click the Button Below

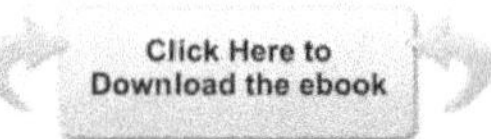

OR **Go to This Page**
http://healthylivingpeople.com/free/

BONUS #2: More Free & Discounted Books or Products
Do you want to receive more Free/Discounted Books or Products?
We have a mailing list where we send out our new Books or Products when they go free or with a discount on Amazon. Click on the link below to sign up for Free & Discount Book & Product Promotions.
=> Sign Up for Free & Discount Book & Product Promotions <=

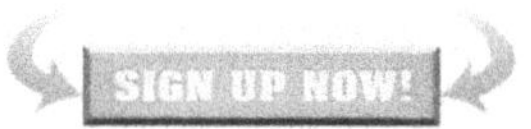

OR Go to this URL
http://zbit.ly/1WBb1Ek